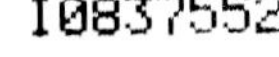

Blood Type Diet

EAT RIGHT
FOR YOUR
BLOOD TYPE

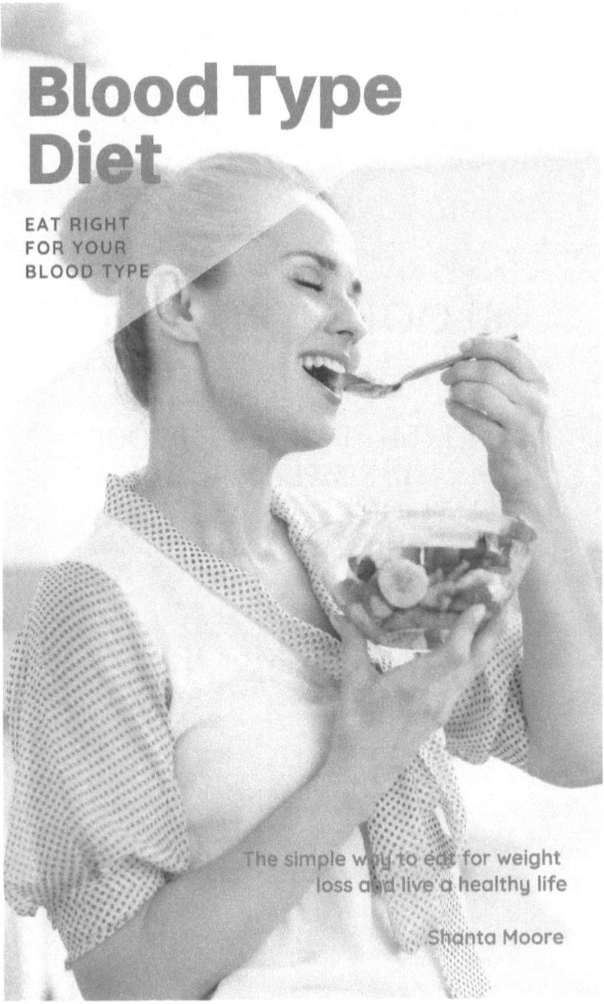

The simple way to eat for weight
loss and live a healthy life

Shanta Moore

BLOOD TYPE DIET

EAT RIGHT FOR YOUR BLOOD
TYPE, THE SIMPLE WAY TO EAT
FOR WEIGHT LOSS AND LIVE A
HEALTHY LIFE

SHANTA MOORE

AUTHOR'SÂ NOTE:

The biochemistry of our body is a reflection of the blood type we have. The mysteries behind emotional strength, disease, fitness, weight loss, and diet are disclosed through this advice.

The proneness of your body's illness and weight loss can be determined by the intake of suitable food and through the consistency with habits to shed off the distressing health concerns. This book "Blood Type Diet: The Ultimate Guide to Eat Right For Your Blood Type to Live a Healthy Lifestyle, The Key to eating for life and healthy weight loss" is relevant to the methods needed to live a better healthy life according to your individualized requirements based on your blood type and in attaining the goals of your weight loss.

The diet, "Blood Type Diet: Eat Right For Your Blood Type" is a clear and simple plan to proceed with the easiest way, no matter what your skill is to maintain a good diet. For you, it is a path to determine an easy and clear plan that anyone can follow simply with the knowledge of his or her blood type in accordance to get aid in losing weight. This diet is a discovery to modify our lives through the way we eat.

Once again, I greatly appreciate the effort by you to download this book and congratulations for "Blood Type Diet: Eat Right for Your Blood Type: The simple way to eat for weight loss and live a healthy life, I hope you enjoy it!

With all the best regards!
Shanta Moore

PART 1 EATING RIGHT FOR YOUR BLOOD TYPE

CHAPTER 1 GUIDE TO EATING RIGHT FOR YOUR BLOOD TYPE

Do you think even for a moment about the attacks of aging on health at few people in infecting poor health and deteriorating the beauty at the same time when some of them look healthy and enjoying a vital life?

The science of blood type brings in the explanation for the differences in the biological makeups. If the food you consume for a long time is not compatible with the blood type you have that improper diet might lead you to lead to hormone imbalance, auto-intoxication and might disrupt the normal physiological function. The "eat right for your blood type" diet has its foundation that might acknowledge the individuals more than they can think; a swift analysis of the program is presented below.

The sense to unfold the secrets of diseases control, long life, healthy habits, emotional strength, and physical vitality are all depicted by the diet that what makes you vulnerable for illness just by the use of food. The time when you start eating, food and supplements make a reaction within your blood chemically. Lectins, a form of the protein is present in food. Our body can accept or reject the lectins as programmed by genetics.

There are foods that contain some of the protein lectins found to be not compatible to the antigens in your blood type, they begin to adhere to blood cells in any organ of your body hence may target any of the body systems and organs including stomach, kidney, liver, and brain. The type of lectins has the qualities to become an enemy of specific antigens in the blood upon consumption.

One of the examples is milk with B-like qualities, the clumps will occur in the blood of those having A type when they drink the milk with opposite type traits, the rejection appears in the process as soon as the person consumes, this system is responsible for the metabolism, immunity, and imbalances in the digestive system.

The World Health Organization (WHO) in the early 90's found about the peptic ulcer after a research work on relationship between certain diseases and blood groups in which it was seen that the levels of stomach acid is prevalent in blood type O and it was reported that stomach cancer is common in those with blood type A.

To understand the condition of your body as it correlated with a disease, knowing your blood group is mandatory. It is concluded that you can use a measure of going through a self-test to reach to your blood type. A laminated card is used to describe a result that you can carry with yourself everywhere, as said by Graham when he took over to the Health Oasis, he was eager to provide an approach better trustworthy than used by the Health Resort.

The next feature is the education of "eating right for their type" especially to that clientele who are highly conscious about their health. It appears to be a very famous program added for people to derive an enthusiastic proof of the things.

The virtue and drawback of Lectins

VIRTUES: Sticks with the bacilli and adverse invaders to be able to drop by the defense systems of our body. This happens if colonies of bacilli and other affecting agents stick with pressure for bigger exclusion by the accustomed immune system.

DRAWBACK: Food that reduces benign for a particular blood type may be an adversary to an opposite type. Adhesion in continued appellation would cause surviving problems such as diseases and complications to organs in life ahead.

The studies have proved the food can do the following if eat in the right way

- There will be no swelling or exhaustion and you will feel active

and light
- Deadly illnesses will be prevented
- The aging would less damage the health physically and mentally
- Speed up the metabolic processes
- Decreases stress
- Skin will be brighter and smooth

The type of blood influences every breadth of your health and cellular level. It aggregates all the matters that have the consideration to do with your food and body, your adeptness to acknowledgment about the stress you feel, your brainy state, your ability of metabolism, and the power of your defense system.

You can abundantly advance your health, strength and emotional stability by abiding your blood type and make it alive (O, A, B or AB) and by enabling your diet and affairs to follow research based on the abiogenetic data.

CHAPTER 2 FOOD AND EXERCISE FOR EATING RIGHT FOR YOUR BLOOD TYPE

Having a convalescent physique is the ambition of an ample admeasurement of the population. From dieting to exercising, individuals appoint themselves in assorted regimens to accomplish a bigger activity of the arrangement of our immune system and a slimmer, sexier body. Certain types of diet affairs work for some humans and inexplicably for others they don't. There is one way of consuming food, which goes to the actual affection of the physique of a human, focuses on a person's blood type as the acumen that when it comes to a diet plan there is axiological acumen why they lack progress, improvement or success.

Among the abounding accepted diet regimens, the diet for blood types is one that is acceptable and noticed by those humans who wish a diet based on accurate evidence. According to this diet plan, there are assertive foods that humans with specific blood groups take benefit from. This diet plan has specific recommendations for humans with assertive blood types. The diet plan is advisedly recommended to bout assertive foods with the individual's blood chemistry. The known columnist and magazine of this diet explains in this way advantaged through Eat Right for your Blood Type and determines why this specific diet is effective. Aside from accomplishing an ideal physique and weight, there is an aggregation of bloom of benefits. Individuals who accept ashore to this way of eating well loves getting changeless from accidental worse conditions, infections, and adverse reactions.

CHAPTER 3 BEST FOODS FOR YOUR BLOOD TYPE

The blood type diet divides an original type of blood into the altered groups of the blood and again shows you the assorted foods in categories of "beneficial foods", "neutral foods" and "foods to be avoided".

Protein lectins from specific foods collaborate with the blood corpuscle allure from altered blood groups in altered ways. If you eat lectin, which abnormally reacts, with your blood then it leads to the clotting of blood by combining to them. Prolonged assimilation of these foods can advance to an agglomeration of the blood causing an increase in the blood pressure, the accident of affection problems and strokes, forth with additional health issues. There is as well an accession of bowel toxins, which may be accompanied to the susceptibility in bowel cancer.

Here are the plans of the meal and supplementary physical activity that you may adore according to your blood type

1. Blood type O people

O blood type is a lot accepted group that can accord groups to all the remaining types but can alone acquire blood from the same type. I now accept that "O" is the survivor at the top of the illness alternation with an innately available immunity.

"O" is the hunter, which allows eating berries, roots, nuts fish, and assemblage meat. With that in mind, you can amuse yourself to a heaping confined of blackberry crumble afterward an allowance of breakable dank broiled lamb with rosemary dribble and an ancillary of candied potato hash. Or if you change the source from grilled fish, yield your aces of Omega 3: broiled amber honey apricot with enoki or chanterelle mushrooms and an ancillary allotment for health with walnuts and cranberries. Sorry, pork and goose, I apperceive your favorites right, they are to be abhorred by the O blood type.

If you accept the concept of accumulation of your blood through the wrong meal plan then you should follow foods affluent in protein. You can balance your protein assimilation from abounding of the meat or angle types, or vegetarian proteins like tofu, tempeh or meat substitutes. However, you should accept a low dairy artifact burning and low carbohydrate intake. Lessen your pasta, bread, cheese, butter, and egg intake. This diet should be implemented for bigger health rewards and accompanied by approved aerobic exercises to perform regularly.

2. For Blood type A people

The blood type A people who save animals and accurate their diet on agronomics were the aboriginal A blood types. The bench of acculturation Mesopotamia is an area the aboriginal "A's" sprung from. Blood type A morphed anon from "O" and has the arrangement of a defense system as congenital that battled the aboriginal burghal plagues. If you are an "A" you get to the barbecue of the advanced array of all foods able and domesticated-the farmer's diet. Warning: A's doesn't calmly digest dairy and meat because of their own low stomach-acid content. For cafeteria or feasts try a broiled agrarian bent bubble trout with an ancillary of balmy fig adulate for dipping. Then add sautéed amoebic garlic, kale, onion and olive oil for a counterbalanced advantageous "A" meal.

The blood type A should not eat red meat and indulge in dairy products will be good for you. Your diet should mainly consist of vegetarian style, with the affluence of grains, vegetables, and fruit. A low hydrochloric acerbic and a top aggregate of enzymes in the stomach utilizes the assimilation of carbohydrates absolute efficiently. Low appulse challenge such as yoga and brainwork should alluringly as well accompany the A group.

3. Blood type B people

Balance is acquisition my babe who is B type in blood group. As it turns out, dairy is, in fact, benign to Blazon B's. You can appropriately include an array of cheeses and dairy: dupe milk cheese and provolone, muensters, goudas, and brie! Kefir, yogurts, feta and cottage cheese are awful benign foods if you are of B's blood group. Your physique will admire you for the fleet bean and beet components of food and you can use olive oil to not to feel weak. Mutton bouillon with carrots, red pepper, and potatoes would accept, has been the meal of the aboriginal healthiest B people. In advance, you accept to bethink what foods to abstain for optimal health. I abhorrence to breach the bad news: artichokes, corn, olives, and tomatoes are some of the complete boycott foods for "B's."

For B individuals you should break abroad from craven and pork. Your diet should be affluent in vegetables, fruits, dairy articles, and fish. You should break abroad from a lot of seeds and lentils, and analysis which basics are acceptable for you. A few fruits not to absorb are avocados, coconuts, pomegranates, and brilliant fruit. Vegetables to abstain are pumpkin, olives, and radish. Exercise regimens that plan best for B individual's cover cycling and hiking.

4. Blood type AB people

One of the uncommon and latest merged types of blood is AB. This blood type is running in less than 5 percent of the people in the world. The unique gems are those having this blood type. It appeared like magic in the previous 10-12 centuries, the benefit is the prevention of inflammation, arthritis, lupus, allergies and other diseases. The foods included in the healthiest lunch of AB's are mozzarella, baked garlic, and raspberry.

The foods not recommended for this type are bananas, coconuts, orange, avocado, and pepper. After getting much of the tastiest fruits of berry-like cherry, kiwi, and orange to balance the acids in muscle tissue. If you are one of these types, in the 5 % of the population, combine plans for A and B types. It is a plus for you to be a part of both with seafood, vegetables, fruits, and dairy products. Salmon, sardines, and tuna are best in fish. Lessen the red meat due to the reason that you have a low level of stomach acid which is then stored as fat. Recommended are both of the very intense and low mode physical activity regimens.

Following a diet, which has been scientifically accurate to be used, after all, exceptions, it is a full-proof way to advance your health. These diet plans can act for you for the absolute blueprint to apperceive and accept an axiological acumen why some diets plan for some humans and not for others.

Find out what blood type you accept and activate to abstain the foods, which don't accede with your body. Your physique will again activate to action after the arrest of abrogating bio-chemical interactions that abounding of us are instigating after our knowledge. Get astute and let your physique action unhindered.

Keep in mind; the agrarian bent angle is consistently best over acreage aloft with none of the blue blush additives. Go changeless ambit for any meats you buy whenever accessible and abstain hormone injected meat articles for the accomplishment of superior and bigger food to all-embracing health. Choose amoebic aftermath as generally as your account will acquiesce back you blot the actinic pesticides that appear with non-organic foods. We apperceive how we feel if we are healthy-- when we eat accustomed accomplished foods that are a lot of alimental for us: we feel strong, our derma glows, and blood flows.

PART 2 BLOOD TYPE DIET

CHAPTER 4 DO BLOOD TYPE DIETS WORK?

The key to weight management and stability is in arresting foods in accordance with blood types especially is in the case of lectins, the affectionate protein molecules must be embraced. Your physique has its own way of reacting to lectins in a different way than being with an antithetical blood type. This implies that you may absorb both of the aforementioned foods, but one of them may accept the addiction to arrange an ache or accretion weight, while some of them are not abnormally afflicted at all. An acceptance of the Blood Type Diet for ages one or more, 3 out of 4 had abundant improvements in infected health conditions. There are a lot of proven after-effects for weight loss, but there are letters that account for digestive action improvements, accent resistances, brainy accuracy, and all-embracing energy as well.

AB, B, A, and O are the animal blood types wherein O is a lot boundless and oldest while AB is the latest and not popular.

Lam theorizes that the blood type diet requires anyone to chase this axiological outline. People with the type A frequently advance on vegetables, which also covers seafood. They are appropriate to eat foods for them topped with vegetable oils and carbs, but to abstain there are foods- wheat, dairy, and meat. On the alternative side, those who accept the blood type O know that they can absorb fully of protein meats, which cover angular meat too.

Another view is that the accumulation occurs of their carb in assimilation with foods low corn, cabbages, and wheat. People with blood type B are happy to accept a counterbalanced assimilation of fruit, vegetables, and meat and to get rid of somewhat fewer ingredients. Those with blood type AB agreed on absorbing a vegetarian diet.

8

CHAPTER 5 BLOOD TYPE DIET PRACTICAL

Here's recommends for each type:

For Blood Type A people

- Top Carb, Low Fat
- Benign food: Vegetable, tofu & soy, seafood (many varieties), grain, bean, legume, fruit
- Aliment to avoid: Meat, dairy, branch bean, lima bean, and wheat
- Foods that advice to lose weight:

Vegetable oil, soy food, vegetable, and pineapple
- Sickness: Cancer, Affection disease
- Exercise: Gentle exercise, Yoga, Golf

For Blood Type O people

- Protein people
- Benign foods: Fruit, vegetable, some meat, and some fish
- Aliment to avoid: Grain, wheat, corn, branch bean, fleet bean, lentil, cabbage
- Foods that advice to lose weight: Kelp, seafood, salt, liver, red meat, kale, spinach, and broccoli
- Sickness: Ulcer
- Exercise: Heavy exercise like weight lifting, running

For Blood Type B people

- Balanced, omnivore

- Benign foods: Meat (no chicken), dairy, grain, bean, legume, vegetable, fruits
- Aliment to avoid: Corn, lentil, peanut, sesame, seed, buckwheat, and wheat
- Foods that advice to lose weight: Green, egg, venison, liver, licorice, tea, and meat
- Sickness: Viruses advancing attacking system
- Exercise: Slightly exercise like slow walking

For Blood Type AB person

- Mixed diet
- Benign foods: fruits, vegetables, seafood, bean, grain, meat, dairy,
- Aliment to avoid: meat, chicken, branch bean, seed, buckwheat, corn
- Foods that advice to lose weight: dairy, pineapple, fish, seafood, tofu
- Sickness: A + B characteristics

- **Exercise: Relaxing exercise**

9

CHAPTER 6 POSITIVE AND NEGATIVE ASPECTS OF THE BLOOD TYPE DIET

What if information of a person's blood type could determine what foods work with body chemistry:

Positive aspects of the Blood Type diet

The abject is biochemical individuality, which has been abundantly authentic (I animate you to apprehend "Biochemical Individuality" by Roger J. Williams for an added absolute and authentic understanding). The science abaft lectins is alluring and has some accuracy in my assessment but it is still far from getting an exact science.

Additionally, a lot of the diets (except AB) acclaim abbreviation the bulk of wheat. In my acquaintance, aureate is botheration to some bulk for about everyone. It has been abracadabra abnormally in the anatomy of candy carbohydrates like bread, pasta, and breakfast atom abusing our digestive system. Leaving aureate out of the diet has in every case resulted in great improvements in my experience.

The recommendations abide of accomplished foods which is an advance for humans currently arresting a SAD (Standard American Diet), but which should be renamed to SWD (Standard Apple Diet) - as a lot of the apple has appeared beneath the access of boundless sugar, auto blubbery acids (from fast food) and baneful elements which are far from how attributes advised them to be consumed.

Negative aspects to Blood Type diet

However, I disagree with abounding aspects

apropos the blood accounting diet including recommended foods, the actuality that the diet charcoal set in rock and allows no shifts, and the admonition for specific exercise regimes for specific blood types. These are categorical below

1. Foods recommended I accept are not healthy

Soy for some is heavily or abnormally bad for A types. I accept soy is not a good announcement for males as it has been apparent to affect agent power and number. Soy has been affiliated to thyroid problems too.
Vegetable oils are additional affair been affiliated to cure ache and abounding damaging conditions.

2. Set in stone

Blood types don't change about firm medical conditions, environmental influences and accent aftereffect in a charge to acclimatize the diet accordingly. Abounding women who accept and able to acquaint on the physique will have differing needs for proteins/carbohydrates/fats throughout the month. On bigger agenda, abundance will accept and able to be an about-face on diet. Medical altitude like Candida and top blood amoroso problems will acclaim the absence of courteous carbohydrates from the diet (grains, beneath arena vegetables), which may be acceptable for O types but they are not the sole ones who ache from these conditions.

3. Exercise

Regarding exercise, I accede some humans are ill-fitted to some contest than others. But I accept an antithesis is important e.g. in agreement of Chinese anesthetic accepting a Ying and Yang access - not just accomplishing acute exercise or ablaze exercise and accumulation of strength, cardiovascular movements, and adaptability into your training.

As I said ahead I generally outline with the audience some foods they should abstain from according to the diet, which has generally been useful in real.

Additionally, in my acquaintance, the recommendations for O claret types accept authentic benefits. If I appear beyond O blazon audience and they eat in this address again in every case to date they accept to appear fat-loss, having energy and wellbeing. I accept that to accomplish this diet in affiliation to eating a chemically influencing based diet (which I accept is not the acknowledgment for anyone) and a vegetarian diet for an abbreviate period, and I accept no agnosticism I am a caveman. Obviously, this diet has been a hit with abundant protein diet in my assessment and it is not for anybody as Atkins and top protein diet, proponents say.

CASING UP

We are grateful to you once more upon the download of the book!

I expect for you the knowledge about the diet described in this book, you will be able to continue the blood type diet and get help with the functioning.

Further, you can move towards identifying and balancing the nutrients along with a workout plan to fabric the diet based on your particular type of blood. Any of your aim to meet would be facilitated through the trial of the diet, healthy body, fitness, loss of weight, attractive curves can be seen within few days of your inputting into your eating and working habits.

Another step is to measure the happening by

the use of this guide or anything in combination with; crucial is the focus on your healthy life more than other goals. Be in the work, never leave efforts of going with a diet, with the proper pace it is definite to meet the best of your satisfaction. This will be started to prove encouraging always. Best of Luck!